Foil Packet Cooking

Delicious Easy Grilled Recipes For Quick Meal, Camping, Outdoor Cooking, Scouting, and Bonfire

Stephanie M. Joseph

TABLE OF CONTENTS

INTRODUCTION

Summer is around the corner and you have planned to go on outdoor camping just to explore the season. Your belief is that a campfire is one of the greatest ways to enjoy your camping.

You have prepared and take stock of what to take along, it remains what and how to take care of your cooking. You have gone on some camping before, but the stress and time you used in washing and cleaning silverware made you reduced the time to explore the park or to engage in other activities that would have made the camping memorable.

You are looking for a method of cooking that will be easy, quick and with less stress, even if your kids are with you in the camp. We are presenting to you an easy, quick, and low-budget way of cooking your meals while on an outdoor camp-Foil packet cooking.

While camping, foil packet meals are the best to enjoy your

adventure.

There is no doubt that foil packet meals are the best ways to go when it comes to eating while camping.

It comes with an easy way to prepare meal- just place the ingredients of the meal on a piece of aluminum foil, wrap it, and place it either in the campfire or on the grill to be cooked.

This method of camp cooking makes the meal to be prepared in few minutes with no problems whatsoever. There are no special tools needed in foil cooking, the essentials tools are a campfire or grill machine, aluminum foil (heavy duty is the best, but if you cannot lay your hands on it, purchase the standard foil from your grocery store, it will work fine), charcoal or wood, fire-resistant gloves, and little time that cannot be compared to the time you use when cooking at home.

There are no scientific rules in starting a campfire to make foil packet meals; build a fire with either wood or charcoal, allow the fire to turn to a bed of hot coals, and place your ingredients in the foil packet on it. Remember that it is only the coals that cook food, while the fire gets it burnt.

Another thing to remember is that while cooking with a foil packet make sure that you are using double-wrapped foil to prevent the steam from getting out of the packet. To achieve this, cut the size of the foil that is big enough to accommodate intended ingredients to be placed at the center. Then cover it with another foil to make it double wrapped. Be sure when folding the packet that it has excess foil around its edges to be able to wrap tightly. It is better to have excess foil than to have not enough foil while wrapping the ingredients.

Before you read more from the book, have these tips at the back of your mind about foil packets:

Make use of heavy-duty foil to prevent burning and tearing of the packet.

Rub butter or cooking oil on the foil to prevent sticking the food to the packet.

Use enough amount of seasonings to make your food more

aroma.

Double fold the packet to keep the moisture in the packet.

Always poke your packet in several parts to allow for heat circulation.

A roaring fire will get your meal burnt-use small fire or white coals and wait until you have a bed of hot coals to have a better meal.

Chapter 1

FOIL-PACKET COOKING

HISTORY OF FOIL-PACKET COOKING

It is not a new thing again finding rolls of aluminum foil in the kitchen cabinets these days, as they are within arm's reach. But, historically aluminum foil was not readily available as a kitchen item as it was originally known as tin. Tin was made in over 100 years and specifically to be used for industrial purposes.

So, in 1910, they replaced the original tin with what is now known as aluminum foil - that was the beginning of food packages in the food industry.

Why the aluminum foil?

The popularity of aluminum foil comes into play with its ability to prevent light, bacterial, and moisture from getting to the food in it. This feature makes it possible for the food to be preserved fresh without been placed in the fridge.

This same feature makes the foil a great way to cook food- just place your ingredients at the center of the foil, make sure the steam in the foil packet is well kept. The steam kept will get the done with moisture and flavor.

What is Aluminum Foil?

Aluminum foil is paper-thin steel of aluminum metal. The aluminum foil is made through rolling slabs of aluminum until they are not up to 0.2mm thick.

Aluminum foil is used for industrial purposes and home used-industrial purposes include food packing, transportation, and insulation. For home use- food storage, wrapping of food, and cooking of food.

Don't be scared of aluminum as we can find it in its natural state in elements such as phosphate, sulfate, air, water in food. You can find it in small amounts in food such as meats, vegetables, grains, fish, and dairy products.

Tools needed for Foil Packet

There are no special tools needed for the foil packet cooking, but listed below are some of the important tools that you may need to bring along when going to the camp with the intention of cooking your meals with aluminum foil.

1. Rotisserie Grill & Spit

If you want your food to be roasted well, go for a rotisserie grill!

This appliance is easy and very convenient to use- make sure to place your foil packet in the middle of it to cook evenly. Remember, as said earlier, wait until you have a bed of hot coals before you place your foiled food.

2. Charcoal Grill

This is an outdoor cooking machine that makes use of charcoal as its fuel source. There are some that come with heat control t, but its main benefit is making the cooking evenly and the meal having a smoky flavor. If you are the type that wants to take part in the grilling of your food; this appliance is your best bet.

3. Grill Gloves

Because you will be handling hot objects while cooking, you will have to get a pair of heat-resistant gloves to save your hands from being burnt. These grill gloves will also give you the confidence of handling spoons, tongs when grilling your food on fire. You have the option of going for the one from hands to arms, or the pair that covers only the hands.

4. Cooking Grate

To have great-looking meals, your foiled packets must be in some distance to the heat. This is just a way to give your food some form of elevation or grate to raise the food above the flames to prevent burning. You may use this grate to boil water or coffee.

It is advised to buy the one with heavy steel as it will prevent oxidation, corrosion, and will withstand any source of heat. The size of it will depend on the number of you that are going camping.

5. Cutting Board

A cutting board is just plywood, plastic, wood, or glass for cutting your ingredients. Buy the one that has a durable surface to cut fruits, vegetables, meat, fish, bread, etc.

6. Water Carrier

If your camping destination is not having water taps or drinking water is not available, it is better to consider carrying a handy water carrier. Your water carrier will give you access to treat the water before use.

7. Knife

Don't forget to pack your knives when you are going camping. Take along different types of knives or multipurpose types of knives that will take care of cutting, chopping, slicing, dicing, peeling, and other tasks required to have delicious meals.

8. Digital Thermometer

Safety comes first!

It will be wrong to come back from camp and be having health related issues because of what you eat while camping. You have to know if what you are cooking is cooked properly. It is this thermometer that you will use to check the right temperatures of what you are cooking. Confirm the temperature of what you are cooking with the standard temperatures as provided by the qualified source.

9. Grill Utensil Set

There are some other grill utensil set that should be with you- spatula, basting brush, tongs, and skewers when you want to have open grilling of fish, meat, fruits, etc.

10. Percolator

If you are a lover of coffee, you may need to bring this utensil along to the camp. This appliance has more benefits than a kettle- as it will make your coffee taste better.

FOOD LIST FOR FOIL PACK COOKING

Eggs	Cinnamon	Tomatoes	Thyme	Olive oil Olives
Green Onions	Balsamic vinegar	Yam	Rosemary	Garlic
Onions	Corn Kernels	Cilantro	Carrots	Sage leaves
Mushrooms	Butter	Water	Green beans	Ginger Root
Potato	Soy Sauce	Peaches	Coconut oil	Coconut
Cheese	Pineapple	Lime	Lemon	Cumin
Sausage	Mint leaves	Chives	Chicken	Turkey
Parsley	Asparagus	Rice	Oregano	Nutmeg
Salt	White wine	Paprika	Salsa	Noodles
Pepper	Almonds	Tarragon	Mayonnaise	Steak
Sour Cream	Pickle relish	Pork	Apricot	Beef
Bacon	Sourdough bread	Coconut milk	Chicken broth	Sriracha Sauce
Avocado	Honey	Hot dogs	Scallions	Shrimp

Muffins	Beer	Fish	Clams	Lobster
Orange	Chocolate bits	Catfish	Trout	Cajun seasoning
Zucchini	Banana	Marshmallow	Crackers	
Red Bell pepper	Whipped cream	Jalapeno pepper	Chili pepper	Ranch dressing
Green bell pepper	Barbecue sauce	Teriyaki sauce	Dijon mustard	Vegetable oil
Taco Seasoning	Jerk seasoning	Worcestershire	Hamburger buns	Alfredo sauce
Apple	Mussels	Oatmeal	Milk	Basil
Sugar	Tortilla	Peanut	Dark Rum	

HOW TO FOLD FOIL PACKET

Remember these tips before you decide to go for foil packet cooking:

1. Buy heavy-duty foil, but if not available go for standard foil as it will also do the magic.

2. Double wrap your ingredients so to prevent the steam from getting out of the packet.

3. Cut more than enough foil for the ingredients. As more than enough is better than not enough.

Back to the folding of the foil to make a packet, cut the foil in large rectangular sheets that will wrap tightly the ingredients to be placed in the center.

There are 2 types of foil packets; the flat foil pack for meal with no liquid, and the one that must make room for food to be steamed.

How to fold the flat-pack, ingredients with no liquid:

Steps:

1. Cut the required size of the foil aluminum, spray the foil with non-sticking oil or spray.

2. Make the size to be more than enough, as less than enough will create a problem later while cooking.

3. Put your entire ingredients at the center of the foil sheet.

4. Wrap the long sides of the foil at the top of the contents and fold it well.

5. Then wrap the foil again and again until the foil is almost at the side of the contents in the foil.

6. Wrap the end of the foil again and again until you are at almost the side of the contents in the foil.

How to fold the tent pack, ingredients with liquid:

Steps:

1. Cut the required size of the foil aluminum, spray the foil with non-sticking oil or spray.

2. Make the size to be more than enough, as less than enough will create a problem later while cooking.

3. Put your entire ingredients at the center of the foil sheet.

4. Pull the long sides of the foil so the two meet at the top, but not seal- making sure they stand upright.

5. Make sure that you double the foil so for the liquid you included among the ingredients will not be drained out.

6. Wrap the short sides many times until you get to almost

the side of the contents in the foil- it will look like an open foil bowl that can hold liquid that was put inside.

7. Wrap the long side down by folding them together again and again until the packet is well sealed.

How to fold foil for steamed food:

Steps:

1. Cut the required size of the foil aluminum, spray the foil with non-sticking oil or spray.

2. Make the size to be more than enough, as less than enough will create a problem later while cooking.

3. Put your entire ingredients at the center of the foil sheet.

4. Raise the long sides of the foil to the top and fold them.

5. Wrap them again and again until you are almost at the side of the contents in the foil.

6. Allow some space between the contents and the foil.

7. Wrap the foil from the ends again and again until you are

almost at the side of the contents in the foil.

Cooking Methods

Below are some common ways to cook your foil packet foods:

Campfire:

Once you have created the campfire, put the packets directly on it, and boom, your food is ready. This method cooks food quickly, but the disadvantage is that the cooking of the food may not be even.

Grill over the campfire:

Grill over the campfire will afford the benefit of not placing your food on the coals directly, as you will make use of grate to elevate it. Because of the reasonable distance between the food and coals, your food will cook evenly.

Barbecue Grill:

Fire the grill, allow it to turn the coals to the bed of hot coals, and put the foil packet on it to be cooked thoroughly. This method affords you the benefit of controlling the temperature of the ingredients you are cooking.

 No matter the type of cooking method you choose, there are some things you have to keep in mind. There is nothing special about campfire as there are lots of factors that will determine the time of cooking for foods.

We advise you to monitor your food well by checking the packet often while cooking to know if the food inside is well cooked. If you open a packet and the food is not well cooked, it is better to return it to the grill to be cooked further.

Remember that some ingredients such as potatoes will take longer time to cook than vegetables like tomatoes, broccoli, and asparagus. So, if you are cooking the three ingredients together, it is better to cut the potatoes into coins or pre-cook to have the three cook properly at the same time.

To add seasonings, herbs, and spices, divide the ingredients in the center and put them inside. But remember that steam will do the cooking. So, adding broth or wine will help in moisture. To make the taste great and delicious, add butter or olive oil.

FOIL PACKET COOKING TIPS

Make use of the following tips when it comes to foil packet cooking:

1. Don't place your packet directly in an open fire- instead, wait until the fire has to turn to the bed of hot coals.

2. Whenever you want to open the packet, open it carefully, as it is full of steam.

3. Make sure to double wrap the ingredients to prevent loss of your food through a hole in the packet's bottom. And you don't want the packet to burst on you while eating.

4. While cooking, check the packet frequently so for the whole packet be evenly cooked.

5. Poke your packet with few holes with the aid of a fork to make the vegetable crisp and a little charred.

6. If you want to eat the food on a plate, cut the top of the packet with a pair of scissors and dump the food on the plate.

7. If you want limited time to cook your food. It is important that you precook some of your ingredients like potatoes, carrots, and celery.

8. Add butter or cooking spray to the ingredients in the foil that do not contain liquid to prevent the sticking of food to the foil.

9. Make sure that you use an internal thermometer to check if your food is cooked properly.

10. Whenever you are cooking food that involves meat or poultry, let them be at the base of the ingredients as they will take more time to cook properly.

11. Whenever you are cooking your fish, let it be in the tent type of foil packet. Add little wine or broth to aid the steaming.

12. Whenever you are cooking your meat, to prevent it from

been dried add a little liquid to aid the steaming.

13. It is important to cut your vegetables into pieces so to reduce the time it will take cooking them properly.

Chapter 2

BREAKFAST RECIPES

Don't start your day with a merry-go-round at the camp without having breakfast in the morning.

Breakfast will surely give you the energy needed to make it through the day even if you don't have time for a lunch meal.

Make sure that you start your day with enough easy and delicious meals in the morning.

SPICED BURRITOS

Ingredients:

2 Eggs

1 Green Onion (small, chopped)

¼ Cup of Onions (chopped)

¼ Cup of Mushrooms (chopped)

1 Potato (small, peeled, cubed)

¾ Cup of Cheese (shredded, blend)

4 oz. of Sausage

¾ Tablespoon of Parsley (fresh, chopped)

Pinch of Salt

Pinch of Pepper

Cilantro

1 Flour Tortilla

Sour Cream

Heavy-Duty Aluminum Foil

Preparation:

1. Break the eggs into a bowl and scramble them.

2. Combine the onion, sausage, mushrooms, potato, cheese, and parsley in the foil packet.

3. Fold the packet at the base and leave the top side open.

4. Top the mixture with the scrambled egg, and then seal it well.

5. Place the packet on the fire to be cooked until the potatoes are soft or for 10 minutes.

6. When the cooking is done, remove from the heat.

7. Pour the cooked content into the tortilla.

8. Use cilantro as garnish and top it with sour cream.

BUTTERED BACON POTATOES

Ingredients:

5 Red Potatoes (baby, sliced)

¼ Cup of Bacon (cooked, crumbled)

1 Tablespoon of Butter

¼ Cup of Mozzarella Cheese

Pinch of Salt

Pinch of Pepper

Heavy-Duty Aluminum Foil

Preparation:

1. Pour the potatoes on the foil packet.

2. Pour the butter on the potatoes, season with salt and pepper; and then lay the bacon on it.

3. Fold the foil tightly to make a packet.

4. Transfer the packet to the heat and cook until potatoes are well cooked or for 15 to 20 minutes.

5. To make the potatoes browned, poke few holes on the foil packet before placing them on the heat.

6. Once the cooking is done, remove from the heat. Open it with care.

7. Add mozzarella to the content in the packet.

8. Open and enjoy.

AVOCADO-EGG BREAKFAST

Ingredients:

1 Avocado (halved, seeded)

2 Eggs

Pinch of Salt

Pinch of Pepper

Heavy-Duty Aluminum Foil

Preparation:

1. Break the eggs into the hollow of the avocado.

2. Place the avocado in two different foil packets and wrap them.

3. Transfer to the heat and cook until the egg is cooked or for 10 to 15 minutes.

4. Unfold the packets carefully; then add salt and pepper.

5. Enjoy.

CHEESY SAUSAGE MUFFIN

Ingredients:

2 Muffins

2 Eggs

2 Sausage patties

2 Hash Brown patties

2 Slices of Cheddar Cheese

Pinch of Salt

Pinch of Pepper

Heavy-Duty Aluminum Foil

Preparation:

1. Put the hash patties in the foil packet, fold and allow the top of it open.

2. Pour the egg on top of the hash brown patties.

3. Place the sausage patties on the egg, and then close the packet.

4. Transfer it to the heat and cook until the egg is done or for 20 to 30 minutes.

5. Remove it from the heat and open the packet.

6. Season it with salt and pepper.

7. Pour the contents inside half of the muffin, top it with cheese, and cover with the other half.

8. Enjoy your sandwich.

Citrus Egg

Ingredients:

1 Orange (meat removed)

2 Eggs

Pinch of Salt

Pinch of Pepper

Heavy-Duty Aluminum Foil

Preparation:

1. Cut the orange into halves and remove the meat inside; make sure the peel remains intact.

2. Break the egg into each half of the orange peel.

3. Wrap each half of the peel with a foil packet; let it be in an upright position so the egg does not spill out.

4. Transfer the packets to the heat and cook until eggs are well cooked or for 15 minutes.

5. Remove from the heat and remove the foil.

6. Season them with salt and pepper.

SPICED SAUSAGE-ZUCCHINI

Ingredients:

2 Sausages (medium, sliced diagonally)

1 Red Bell pepper (seeded, sliced)

1 Zucchini (sliced diagonally)

1 Onion (small, sliced)

Pinch of Salt

Pinch of Pepper

Heavy-Duty Aluminum Foil

Preparation:

1. Mix the entire ingredients in a foil packet.

2. Cover the foil packet tightly.

3. Place the packet on the heat and cook until the veggies are soft or for 20 to 30 minutes.

4. Remove from the heat and enjoy.

SEASONED CHEESY GRILLED BEEF

Ingredients:

8 oz. of Carne Asada

2 Eggs

2 Tablespoons of Taco seasoning

½ Cup of Cheddar Cheese

Heavy-Duty Aluminum Foil

Preparation:

1. Cut the grilled beef and place it in the packet.

2. Season it with taco and pour the egg on it.

3. Make sure that the egg rubs the beef well.

4. Place the packet on the heat and cook until the beef and egg are thoroughly cooked or for 15 to 20 minutes.

5. When done open one side of the packet and sprinkle cheese on top of it.

6. You can eat it all alone or add it to a tortilla for a delicious breakfast.

CHEESY BACON MUFFIN

Ingredients:

1 Slice of Ham (cooked)

1 Muffin

1 Egg

1 Slice of Bacon (cooked)

Heavy-Duty Aluminum Foil

1 Slice of Pepper jack cheese

Preparation:

1. Put the muffin in the center of the foil packet.

2. Put bacon and ham on top of the muffin.

3. Top it with egg and cover the packet and leave part of one side of the packet open.

4. Cook until the egg is cooked or for 10 to 15 minutes; remove from the heat and top it with cheese.

5. Enjoy.

EGG & ONION

Ingredients:

2 Eggs

1 medium Onion (sliced)

Heavy-Duty Aluminum Foil

Preparation:

1. Mold 2 cups with foil aluminum; make the bottom 1 lb. and 3 inches in diameter.

2. Break an egg into each cup and add sliced onions.

3. Transfer the cups to the heat and cook until the eggs are cooked or for 10 to 15 minutes.

4. Enjoy.

Chapter 3

FRUIT & VEGGIES

Aluminum foil is one of the best ways to cook fruits and veggie meals. There is no technical way than to simply pour your ingredients in the foil packet, add spices, and season it to make it taste great. Next is to transfer the packet to the fire and wait for as little as 10 to 40 minutes and your meal is ready to be consumed.

SWEET APPLE PIE

Ingredients:

2 Apples (any color)

2 Tablespoons of Brown sugar

½ Cup of Apple pie filling

2 Tablespoons of Cinnamon

1 Pie crust (rolled)

Heavy-Duty Aluminum Foil

Preparation:

1. Use a knife to cut the top of the apples.

2. Scoop out the inside of the apples to make room in the apples.

3. Combine cinnamon, apple pie filling, and brown sugar in a bowl.

4. Use a spoon to pour the mix into the apples, and then pour the pie crust on top of it.

5. Place the apple on the foil and make it tightly with the fruit.

6. Transfer the packet to the heat and cook until the crust begins to turn brown and the filling is hot or for 20 to 25 minutes.

Spiced Vinegar Balsamic

Ingredients:

2 Tomatoes (halved)

Pinch of thyme (dried)

3 Tablespoons of Olive oil

2 Teaspoons of Balsamic vinegar

Pinch of Salt

Pinch of Pepper

Heavy-Duty Aluminum Foil

Preparation:

1. Place the tomatoes halves on the foil face up.

2. Pour the olive oil on it, and sprinkle dried thyme on the tomatoes.

3. Then drizzle vinegar on the tomatoes.

4. Use salt and pepper to season it.

5. Wrap the contents in the foil tightly to make a packet.

6. Transfer the packet to the heat and cook until well cooked or for 30 to 40 minutes.

ROSEMARY YAMS

Ingredients:

2 Tablespoons of Thyme (fresh)

2 Pounds of Yam (peeled, sliced)

2 Sprigs of Rosemary

2 Green Onions (sliced)

2 cloves of Garlic (minced)

¼ Cup of Olive oil

Pinch of Salt

Pinch of Pepper

Heavy-Duty Aluminum Foil

Preparation:

1. Combine the entire ingredients in a foil packet well.

2. Wrap the contents in the foil tightly to make a packet.

3. Make several pokes on the top side of the packet.

4. Transfer the packet to the heat and cook until the yams are well cooked or for 15 to 20 minutes.

5. Enjoy.

Creamy Bacon Corn

Ingredients:

2 Cups of Corn Kernels

½ Cup of Cheese (shredded)

½ Cup of Onions (chopped)

1 Cup of Sour Cream

1 Cup of Bacon (crumbled)

1 Tablespoon of Cilantro (chopped)

Heavy-Duty Aluminum Foil

Preparation:

1. Combine the entire ingredients in a small bowl.

2. Divide the mix into two foil packets, and then wrap them tightly.

3. Transfer the packets to the heat and cook for 5 minutes.

4. Flip them over and continue cooking for another 3 minutes.

5. Open them carefully and serve while warm.

BUTTERED SAGE & CARROTS

Ingredients:

1 Cup of Carrots (cut into pieces)

1 Clove of Garlic (chopped)

1 ½ Teaspoons of Sage leaves

½ Tablespoon of Butter

1 Tablespoon of Water

½ Teaspoon of Olive oil

Heavy-Duty Aluminum Foil

Preparation:

1. Combine the entire ingredients in a foil packet except for sage leaves.

2. Wrap the packet and allow room at the top for heat circulation.

3. Transfer the packet to the heat and cook until carrots are soft or for 10 minutes.

4. Remove from the heat; then open it and sprinkle sage leave to garnish.

GINGER BEANS SAUCE

Ingredients:

1 Cup of Green beans

½ Teaspoons of Ginger root (ground)

1 clove of Garlic (minced)

2 Tablespoons of Soy sauce

1 Tablespoon of Brown sugar

1 Tablespoon of Butter (melted)

Pinch of Salt

Pinch of Pepper

Heavy-Duty Aluminum Foil

Preparation:

1. Add the entire ingredients in a foil packet except for salt

and pepper.

2. Wrap up the packet and allow the top of the packet to open for heat circulation.

3. Transfer to the heat and cook until green beans are cooked well or for 10 minutes.

4. Open the packet and add salt and pepper.

Sweet Creamy Peaches

Ingredients:

2 Peaches (halved, pitted)

2 Tablespoons of Coconut oil

½ Cup of Whipped cream

2 Tablespoons of Cinnamon

2 Tablespoons of Sugar (granulated)

2 Tablespoons of Honey

Heavy-Duty Aluminum Foil

Preparation:

1. Use a knife to cut the peaches into halves, and then place them on the packet side up.

2. Pour the coconut oil on top of the peaches.

3. Spray the sugar on top of the peaches.

4. Turn the peaches side down and wrap the packet up tightly.

5. Transfer the packet to the heat and cook for 3 minutes; then flip to the other side and cook for another 3 minutes.

6. Open the packet and turn the peaches over.

7. Add cinnamon to it and drizzle honey on it.

8. Top the peaches with whipped cream.

SPICED GRILLED POTATOES

Ingredients:

1 Potato (big, cubed)

2 Tablespoons of Parsley

1 Tablespoon of Olive oil

¼ Onion (diced)

2 Tablespoons of Rosemary

1 clove of Garlic (minced)

1 Teaspoon of Oregano

Pinch of Salt

Pinch of Pepper

Heavy-Duty Aluminum Foil

Preparation:

1. Add the entire ingredients in a small bowl thoroughly.

2. Pour the contents on a foil and tight it well to make a packet.

3. Transfer the packet to the heat and cook until the potatoes are well cooked or for 20 to 30 minutes.

4. Flip the packet over to the other side and cook for another 10 minutes.

5. Enjoy.

Peppery Olives

Ingredients:

1 Can of Olives (drained)

2 cloves of Garlic (minced)

1 Teaspoon of Red pepper flakes

Heavy-Duty Aluminum Foil

Preparation:

1. Pour the olives on a foil.

2. Add garlic and pepper flakes to it.

3. Mix the contents well in the packet.

4. Then wrap up the foil tightly to make a packet and allow room for heat circulation.

5. Transfer the packet to the heat and cook until the olives

are heated well or for 10 to 15 minutes.

SPICED JALAPENO

Ingredients:

4 Jalapeno peppers (halved, deseeded)

1 Cup of Cheddar cheese

2 Tablespoons of Olive oil

½ Teaspoon of Cumin

1 Teaspoon of Salt

Pinch of Coriander

Heavy-Duty Aluminum Foil

Preparation:

1. Mix coriander, olive oil, cumin, and salt in a small bowl.

2. Spoonful the coriander mix into the jalapeno halves; then place them upright on the foil packet.

3. Create a foil packet that has enough room for steam.

4. Transfer the packet to the heat and grill until the jalapenos are soft and cheese is melted.

5. Serve and enjoy.

Sour Creamy Baked Potato

Ingredients:

2 Potatoes (small, baked)

3 Tablespoons of Sour cream

2 Tablespoons of Butter

1 Green onion (chopped)

1 Cup of Cheddar cheese (shredded)

3 Tablespoons of Bacon bits

Heavy-Duty Aluminum Foil

Preparation:

1. Put the baked potatoes on the foil.

2. Rub the butter on the potatoes, and then add cheese, green onion, and bacon to it

3. Wrap the foil tightly to make a packet; then poke it severally with a fork.

4. Transfer the packet to heat and cook until the potatoes are soft.

5. Open the packet and remove the potatoes; then add sour cream to taste.

Mayo Corn

Ingredients:

1 Corn

1 Lime (wedged)

2 Tablespoons of Mayonnaise

2 Tablespoons of Cheddar cheese (crumbled)

½ clove of Garlic (minced)

½ Teaspoon of Salt

½ Teaspoon of Chili pepper

Heavy-Duty Aluminum Foil

Preparation:

1. Combine mayonnaise, salt, garlic, and chili pepper in a small bowl.

2. Rub the mayo mix on the corn and then place it on a foil.

3. Wrap the foil tightly to make a packet.

4. Transfer the packet to the heat and cook until the corn is cooked or for 20 to 25 minutes.

5. Remove from the heat, and rub the corn again with mayo mix.

6. Rub the crumbled cheese on the corn.

7. Enjoy.

GRILLED SNAP PEAS

Ingredients:

1 Cup of Snap peas (end broken)

1 Tablespoon of Olive oil

3 Tablespoons of Mint leaves (chopped)

Pinch of Salt

Heavy-Duty Aluminum Foil

Preparation:

1. Combine olive oil and salt in a bowl.

2. Add peas to the mixture in a bowl.

3. Put the peas on a foil and wrap to make a packet, allow room for the circulation of heat.

4. Transfer the packet to heat and cook until peas begin to soften.

5. Open the packet and add mint.

6. Serve and enjoy.

Creamy Chives Potatoes

Ingredients:

5 Potatoes (small, sliced)

½ Tablespoon of Olive oil

2 Tablespoons of Sour cream

1 ½ Tablespoons of Water

3 Tablespoons of Yogurt (plain)

½ Teaspoon of Chives

Pinch of Salt

Pinch of pepper

Heavy-Duty Aluminum Foil

Preparation:

1. Combine sour cream, chives, and yogurt in a small bowl.

2. Pour the potatoes on a foil, and then drizzle oil over it.

3. Add salt and pepper.

4. Wrap the foil tightly to make a packet and open-top side of the packet.

5. Pour in water and allow room for the circulation of heat.

6. Transfer the packet to the heat and cook until the potatoes are soft or for 20 to 25 minutes.

7. Remove it from the heat and carefully open it.

8. Pour the sour cream mix on top of the potatoes.

CHEESY ZUCCHINI

Ingredients:

2 Zucchini (sliced)

2 Tablespoons of Butter (melted)

2 cloves of Garlic

½ Cup of Parmesan cheese

Pinch of Salt

Pinch of Pepper

Heavy-Duty Aluminum Foil

Preparation:

1. Put the zucchini and garlic on a foil.

2. Pour the melted butter on top of the zucchini and garlic.

3. Season it with salt and pepper to taste.

4. Fold the foil tightly to make a packet, and allow room for heat circulation.

5. Transfer it to the heat and cook until the zucchini and garlic begin to soft or for 20 to 25 minutes.

6. Remove it from the heat and carefully open it.

7. Pour the parmesan cheese on top of the zucchini and garlic.

8. Return the packet to the heat and cook again for another 3 to 5 minutes while the packet is opened.

Sweet Roasted Garlic

Ingredients:

5 cloves of Garlic

¼ Cup of Olive oil

Pinch of Salt

Pinch of Pepper

Heavy-Duty Aluminum Foil

Preparation:

1. Put the garlic on a foil.

2. Rub them with olive oil.

3. Add salt and pepper to taste.

4. Cover the foil tightly to make the packet.

5. Transfer the packet to the heat and cook until garlic cloves

are well roasted.

3. Serve and enjoy.

Sweet Rosemary Potatoes

Ingredients:

5 Potatoes (sliced)

¼ Sweet onion (sliced)

½ Teaspoon of Rosemary (fresh, chopped)

3 Tablespoons of Olive oil

Pinch of Salt

Pinch of Pepper

Heavy-Duty Aluminum Foil

Preparation:

1. Put the potatoes and onions on a foil.

2. Coat them with olive oil, and fold the foil to make a packet.

3. Then fold it tightly to make a packet.

4. Transfer the packet to the heat and cook until the potatoes are well cooked or for 15 to 15 minutes.

5. Turn the packet to the other side and cook for another 10 minutes.

6. Remove from the heat open carefully, and garnish with rosemary.

7. Add salt and pepper to taste.

Buttered Corn

Ingredients:

2 Sweet corns

2 Tablespoons of Butter

Pinch of Salt

Pinch of Pepper

Heavy-Duty Aluminum Foil

Preparation:

1. Rub the melted butter on the corns.

2. Season the buttered corns with salt and pepper.

3. Place the corn on the foil; Fold the foil tightly to make a packet.

4. Transfer the packet to the heat and cook for 15 to 20

minutes.

5. Make sure to flip every 3 minutes.

6. Remove the packet from the heat and open it carefully.

7. Enjoy.

Bacon Swiss Chard

Ingredients:

1 Cup of Swiss chard (leaves only)

1 Tablespoon of Butter

¼ Cup of Bacon bits

1 clove of Garlic (minced)

Pinch of Salt

Pinch of Pepper

Heavy-Duty Aluminum Foil

Preparation:

1. Pour the chard leaves on a foil; rub with butter.

2. Add bacon bit and garlic on it and.

3. Season it with salt and pepper to taste.

4. Fold the foil tightly to make a packet, and allow room for heat circulation.

5. Transfer to the heat and cook until the leaves are wilt but not completely cook or for 3 to 5 minutes.

6. Carefully open the packet and enjoy.

BREADCRUMB STUFFED PEPPERS

Ingredients:

2 Bell pepper (deseeded, halved)

½ Pound of Turkey (ground)

¼ Cup of Garlic (powder)

½ Onion (diced)

1 Teaspoon of Salt

1 Teaspoon of Pepper

1/3 Cup of Breadcrumbs (crushed)

Preparation:

1. Blend turkey, garlic powder, onion, breadcrumbs, salt, and pepper in a bowl with hands.

2. Use your hands to fill the bell peppers with the turkey mix;

and then place the filled peppers face down on a foil.

3. Fold the foil tightly to make a packet.

4. Transfer the packet to the heat and cook for 25 to 35 minutes.

5. Turn the packet halfway while cooking.

6. When the peppers are soft and the turkey is well cooked the cooking is done.

Sour Feta & Tomatoes

Ingredients:

10 Cherry Tomatoes

1 clove of Garlic (chopped)

¾ Cup of Feta cheese

¼ Cup of Balsamic vinegar

2 Tablespoons of Olive oil

Heavy-Duty Aluminum Foil

Preparation:

1. Put the tomatoes on foil.

2. Pour the feta cheese to cover it, and then add garlic on top.

3. Drizzle vinegar and olive oil on it.

4. Fold the foil tightly to make a packet; then allow room for

the circulation of heat.

5. Transfer to the heat and cook until the tomatoes are well cooked or for 15 to 20 minutes.

6. Enjoy.

Baked Onion-Tomatoes

Ingredients:

5 Cherry Tomatoes (firm, halved crosswise)

1 Sweet onion (sliced)

Pinch of Salt

Pinch of Pepper

Heavy-Duty Aluminum Foil

Preparation:

1. Sprinkle the tomato halves with salt and pepper.

2. Put the onion slices in between the tomatoes and hold with toothpicks.

3. Rub the foil with butter to make it non-sticking.

4. Place the filled tomatoes on a foil; then fold them

individually to make different packets.

5. Transfer to the heat and cook for 15 to 20 minutes.

6. Enjoy.

Creamy Green Beans

Ingredients:

16 oz. of Green Beans (drained)

3 Tablespoons of Cream cheese

Heavy-Duty Aluminum Foil

Preparation:

1. Rub the foil with non-sticking oil.

2. Mix cheese with beans in a small bowl.

3. Put the mixture at the center of the foil and add salt and pepper.

4. Wrap the foil tightly to make a packet.

5. Transfer to the heat and cook for 15 to 20 minutes.

Sweet Grilled Squash

Ingredients:

2 Acorn Squash (halved, deseeded)

1 Tablespoon of Margarine

1 Tablespoon of Water

1 Tablespoon of Brown sugar

1 Apple (peeled, wedged)

Heavy-Duty Aluminum Foil

Preparation:

1. Use a fork to dig inside of squash; then add salt and pepper.

2. Add 1 teaspoon of sugar, margarine, and water to each squash half; then top it with apple pieces.

3. Fold each of the squash sides up to make a packet.

4. Transfer the squash side up on the heat and cook until the squash is cooked or for 35 to 45 minutes

.

Chapter 4

CHICKEN & TURKEY RECIPES

All the dishes in this section involve chicken and turkey in one form or another.

It is important to remember that whenever you want to cook chicken and turkey, it has to be cooked thoroughly- meaning there must not be any pink on the meat, and the juices coming out must be clear when you cut the meat into pieces.

CREAMY MUSHROOM CHICKEN

Ingredients:

4 Pieces of Chicken

1 Cup of Cream chicken soup

1 ½ Cups of Asparagus (pieces)

1 Cup of Mushrooms (sliced)

Heavy-Duty Aluminum Foil

Preparation:

1. Put the chicken on a foil, and lay the mushrooms and asparagus around the chicken.

2. Pour the chicken soup over the contents.

3. Fold the foil tightly to make a packet, allowing room for heat circulation.

4. Transfer the packet to the heat and cook until the chicken is well cooked or for 30 to 40 minutes.

Spiced Herbed Chicken

Ingredients:

1 Chicken breasts

½ Cup of Rice (cooked)

½ Cup of Broccoli

Pinch of Oregano

½ Cup of Mushroom soup (cream)

Pinch of Paprika

½ Teaspoon of Garlic (powder)

Pinch of Salt

Pinch of Pepper

Heavy-Duty Aluminum Foil

Preparation:

1. Piece the chicken breast into bits.

2. Place the bits on a foil and add other ingredients around the chicken.

3. Fold the foil tightly to make a packet, allowing room for heat circulation.

4. Transfer the packet to the heat and cook until the chicken is well cooked and broccoli is softened or for 30 to 40 minutes.

DRESSED BACON CHICKEN

Ingredients:

1 Chicken breast (skinless, boneless, cubed)

4 Slices of Bacon (cooked, pieces)

1 Cup of Cheddar cheese

2 Tablespoons of Olive oil

2 Tablespoons of Ranch Dressing

Heavy-Duty Aluminum Foil

Preparation:

1. Rub the olive oil on the chicken pieces and lay on a foil.

2. Pour ranch dressing on the chicken, and then place cheese on top of it.

3. Sprinkle the cooked bacon on top of the cheese.

4. Then fold the foil tightly to make a packet.

5. Transfer the packet to the heat and cook until the chicken is well cooked or for 20 to 30 minutes.

6. Enjoy.

Buttered Potatoes & Chicken

Ingredients:

1 Chicken breast (cubed)

½ Cup of Barbecue sauce

2 Potatoes (medium, cubed, not peeled)

1 Teaspoon of Salt

2 Tablespoons of Butter

½ Teaspoon of Black pepper

Heavy-Duty Aluminum Foil

Preparation:

1. Pour the potatoes on a foil.

2. Then pour half of the butter on it.

3. Fold the foil tightly to make a packet, and place it on the heat.

4. Cook until the potatoes begin to turn brown or for 15 to 20 minutes.

5. Open the packet and add the remaining ingredients.

6. Cover the packet back and return to the heat to be cooked for an additional 15 to 20 minutes or until the chicken is well cooked.

Dressed Bean & Chicken

Ingredients:

1 Chicken breast

½ Cup of Green beans (fresh, ends removed)

2 Red potatoes (sliced)

8 Black olives (sliced)

4 Cherry Tomatoes

3 Tablespoons of Ranch dressing

Heavy-Duty Aluminum Foil

Preparation:

1. Lay the chicken on a foil.

2. Rub the dressing on the chicken, and then add veggies around it.

3. Fold the foil tightly to make a packet, allowing room for heat circulation.

4. Transfer the packet to the heat and cook until the chicken is well cooked and the veggies are soft or for 20 to 30 minutes.

CHICKEN & TERIYAKI SAUCE

Ingredients:

1 Chicken breast (boneless, skinless)

1 Red pepper (sliced)

½ Cup of Pineapple chunks (drained)

½ Cup of Teriyaki sauce

Heavy-Duty Aluminum Foil

Preparation:

1. Put the entire ingredients on foil.

2. Wrap the foil tightly to make a packet, allowing room for heat circulation.

3. Transfer the packet to the heat and cook until the chicken is well cooked or for 20 to 30 minutes.

4. Turn the packet to the other side and cook for additional
10 minutes.

Spiced Sweet Chicken

Ingredients:

2 Chicken wings

3 cloves of Garlic (minced)

¼ Cup of Allspice

2 Tablespoons of Olive oil

¼ Cup of Brown sugar

1 Tablespoon of Thyme (ground)

½ Teaspoon of Cinnamon

1 Teaspoon of Onion (minced, dried)

½ Teaspoon of Nutmeg

2 Bonnet peppers

Heavy-Duty Aluminum Foil

Preparation:

1. Pour the entire ingredients in a food processor, except chicken; then pulse until all well puree.

2. Put the chicken wings in a plastic bag and pour the pureed on it; allow to marinate for few hours.

3. Remove the chicken from the bag and lay it on a foil.

4. Pour the remaining purred on it.

5. Transfer the packet to the heat and cook until the chicken is well cooked or for 20 to 30 minutes.

6. Turn the packet to the other side and cook for additional 15 minutes.

CHEESY POTATOES & CHICKEN

Ingredients:

2 Chicken breasts

4 Red Potatoes (quartered)

1 Cup of Spaghetti sauce

1 Onion (small, diced)

1/3 Cup of Parmesan cheese

Heavy-Duty Aluminum Foil

Preparation:

1. Lay the chicken on a foil.

2. Place potatoes and onions around the chicken.

3. Pour sauce on top of it; then spray the Parmesan on top.

4. Wrap the foil tightly to make a packet.

5. Transfer the packet to the heat and cook until the chicken is well cooked and potatoes are soft or for 20 to 30 minutes.

6. Enjoy.

MUSTARD CHICKEN

Ingredients:

2 Chicken breasts (boneless, pounded)

1 Jalapeno pepper (sliced)

1 Cup of Mixed peppers (green, yellow, red, cut into strips)

1 Teaspoon of Salt

1 Teaspoon of Butter

¼ Cup of White wine

2 Tablespoons of Dijon Mustard

Heavy-Duty Aluminum Foil

Preparation:

1. Blend wine, butter, mustard, and salt in a bowl well.

2. Use the mixture to rub the chicken.

3. Put the pepper strips around the chicken on a foil.

4. Wrap the chicken around peppers and hold it securely with wooden picks.

5. Wrap the foil tightly to make a packet.

6. Transfer the packet to the heat and cook until the chicken is well cooked and the peppers are soft or for 20 to 30 minutes.

Delicious BBQ Chicken

Ingredients:

5 Chicken Wings

¼ Cup of Barbecue sauce

Pinch of Salt

¼ Cup of Hot sauce

Pinch of Pepper

Ranch dressing

Heavy-Duty Aluminum Foil

Preparation:

1. Combine hot sauce, barbecue sauce, salt, and pepper in a big bowl well.

2. Put the chicken in the bowl and stir until chicken wings are well coated with the sauce.

3. Remove the coated wings and place them on a foil; then pour the sauce over the wings.

4. Wrap the foil tightly to make a packet; making sure the wings are in a straight line on the foil before wrapping.

5. Transfer the packet to the heat and cook until the chicken is well cooked or for 20 to 30 minutes.

6. Serve while warm with ranch dressing.

PEPPERY SPICED CHICKEN

Ingredients:

1 Pound Chicken breasts (skinless, boneless, cut into strips)

2 Red bell peppers (sliced)

2 Green bell peppers (sliced)

1 Onion (chopped)

2 Jalapeno pepper (sliced)

10 Olives (sliced)

2 Teaspoons of Salt

½ Teaspoons of Cayenne pepper

Heavy-Duty Aluminum Foil

Preparation:

1. Combine the entire ingredients on a foil well.

2. Wrap the foil tightly to make a packet, allowing room for heat circulation.

3. Transfer the packet to the heat and cook until the chicken is well cooked or for 20 to 30 minutes.

Cheesy Zucchini Chicken

Ingredients:

1 Zucchini (medium, halved)

1 Pound of Turkey (ground)

½ Teaspoon of Paprika

1 Teaspoon of Cumin

1 Cup of Salsa

¼ Cup of Tomato sauce

½ Teaspoon of Salt

2 Tablespoons of Bell pepper (diced)

½ Teaspoon of Oregano

½ Teaspoon of Garlic powder

Cheddar cheese

Heavy-Duty Aluminum Foil

Preparation:

1. Create a deep trench with a spoon in the halves of zucchini.

2. Mix garlic, cumin, oregano, salt, and paprika in a bowl well.

3. Blend turkey, tomato sauce, and bell pepper in another bowl well.

4. Mix the two bowls together and make sure the turkey is well coated with the sauce.

5. Place the zucchini halves on the foil.

6. Use a spoon to fill the trenches of the zucchini halves with the turkey filling; make sure that the trenches are well filled.

7. Sprinkle the cheese on top of the zucchini halves.

8. Wrap the foil tightly to make a packet; then poke severally the top of the packet.

9. Transfer the packet to the heat and cook until the zucchini halves begin to soften or for 25 to 35 minutes.

10. Enjoy.

PINEAPPLE & CHICKEN

Ingredients:

2 Chicken breast (skinless, boneless)

¼ Cup of Sour sauce

¼ Cup of Chow mein noodles

½ Bell pepper (strips)

¼ Onion (wedged)

4 oz. of Pineapple chunks (drained)

Heavy-Duty Aluminum Foil

Preparation:

1. Place the chicken on a foil and pour sauce, pineapple chunks, pepper strips, and onion wedges on it.

2. Wrap the foil tightly to make a packet.

3. Transfer the packet to the heat, cook turn it every 5 minutes until done or for 20 to 25 minutes.

4. Open the packet carefully and pour it on top of the noodles.

5. Serve and enjoy.

Jerk Seasoned Chicken

Ingredients:

3 Chicken wings

Tablespoons of Jerk seasoning

2 Tablespoons of Cilantro (chopped)

1 Tablespoon of Vegetable oil

3 Lemon wedges

Heavy-Duty Aluminum Foil

Preparation:

1. Mix vegetable oil and jerk seasoning in a bowl; then use the mixture to coat the wings.

2. Put the coated wings on a foil and pour the remaining mix on it.

3. Wrap the foil tightly to make a packet.

4. Transfer the packet to the heat, cook turn it every 10 minutes until done or for 20 to 25 minutes.

5. When the cooking is done, add cilantro and serve with a lemon wedge.

Worcestershire Chicken

Ingredients:

2 Chicken breast (skinless, boneless, pieces into bits)

2 Teaspoons of Worcestershire

4 Cherry tomatoes

2 Potatoes (peeled, cuts)

2 Slices of Onion

4 Green pepper rings (sliced)

2 Tablespoons of Butter

4 Mushrooms (large, sliced)

Pinch of Paprika

Pinch of Salt

Pinch of Pepper

Heavy-Duty Aluminum Foil

Preparation:

1. Place the chicken pieces on a foil and pour on top of it the remaining ingredients.

2. Wrap the foil tightly to make a packet.

3. Transfer the packet to the heat, cook until the chicken is opaque and the potatoes are soft or for 25 to 35 minutes.

4. Enjoy.

SWEET LEMONY CHICKEN

Ingredients:

2 Chicken breast (bone-in)

2 Tablespoons of Butter

2 Tablespoons of Onion (chopped)

2 Tablespoons of Brown sugar

½ Teaspoon of Salt

½ Teaspoon of Mustard (dried)

2 Tablespoons of Lemon juice

Heavy-Duty Aluminum Foil

Preparation:

1. Pour the butter in a skillet and brown the chicken slightly; then sauté onions in the same skillet.

2. Sprinkle the sautéed onion on the chicken.

3. Combine sugar, salt, mustard, and pepper in a bowl.

4. Pour the mustard mix in a bowl over the chicken placed on a foil; then pour the remaining sautéed oil in the skillet over the chicken.

5. Wrap the foil tightly to make a packet.

6. Transfer the packet to the heat, cook until the chicken is well cooked or for 25 to 35 minutes.

Oriental Pine Chicken

Ingredients:

2 Chicken breasts (bone-in)

½ Cup of Almonds

2 Slices of Pineapple (drained)

Pinch of Salt

Pinch of Pepper

Pinch of Tarragon

Pinch of Rosemary

Heavy-Duty Aluminum Foil

Preparation:

1. Pour the butter in a skillet and brown the chicken slightly; then sauté pineapple and almonds in the same skillet.

2. Sprinkle the sautéed ingredients on the chicken placed on a foil.

3. Then add rosemary, tarragon, salt, and pepper to it.

4. Wrap the foil tightly to make a packet.

5. Transfer the packet to the heat, cook until the chicken is well cooked or for 25 to 35 minutes.

6. Enjoy.

MAYO HAMBURGER CHICKEN

Ingredients:

2 Chicken breasts (chopped)

3 Green olives (chopped)

¼ Cup of Mayonnaise

1 Egg (hard-boiled, chopped)

1 Tablespoon of Pickle relish

6 Hamburger buns (small)

1 Tablespoon of Onion (chopped)

½ Cup of Cheese (cubed)

Heavy-Duty Aluminum Foil

Preparation:

1. Combine the entire ingredients in a bowl well.

2. Divide the mixture into two, and pour them into different foils

3. Wrap the foils tightly to make packets.

4. Transfer the packets to the heat, cook until the chicken is well cooked or for 15 to 20 minutes.

5. Enjoy.

DELIGHT SWEET CHICKEN

Ingredients:

2 Chicken breasts (bone-in, skinless)

2 Tablespoons of Margarine

Pinch of Salt

Pinch of Pepper

Heavy-Duty Aluminum Foil

Preparation:

1. Rub butter, salt, and pepper on the chicken.

2. Place the chicken breasts on different foils, making sure the ribs are side up.

3. Wrap the foils tightly to make packets.

4. Transfer the packets to the heat, cook until the chicken is

well cooked or for 20 to 30 minutes.

5. Enjoy.

Grilled Potatoes Zucchini Chicken

Ingredients:

3 Chicken breast (bone-in)

3 Carrots (halved lengthwise)

3 Tablespoons of Onion mix soup

3 Potatoes (medium, peeled, quartered)

1 Cup of Zucchini

1 Can of Cream chicken soup (diluted with water)

Heavy-Duty Aluminum Foil

Preparation:

1. Put the chicken in three different foils.

2. Then divide the vegetables among the three chickens.

3. Pour the onion soup mix on them and drizzle chicken soup diluted with ½ cup of water on top.

4. Transfer the packets to the heat, and grill until the chicken is well cooked or for 30 to 40 minutes.

5. Enjoy.

Chapter 5

PORK & BEEF RECIPES

The recipes in this section are some of the delicious meals that come from pork and beef while camping. They are easy and quick to be prepared. Relax and get your hands dirty a bit while eating your favorite meals.

BUTTERED PORK CHOP

Ingredients:

2 Pork chops

2 Tablespoons of Butter (melted)

1 ½ Cups of Apricot

2 Teaspoons of Balsamic vinegar

Heavy-Duty Aluminum Foil

Preparation:

1. Blend apricot, butter, and vinegar in a small bowl well.

2. Coat each pork with the mix in the bowl.

3. Put the pork chops in two different foils.

4. Pour the remaining mix on top of the pork chops.

5. Fold the foils tightly to make packets.

6. Transfer the packets to the heat and cook until the pork chops are well cooked or for 15 to 20 minutes.

7. Enjoy.

CHEESY BACON HAMBURGERS

Ingredients:

2 Hamburger Patties

4 Slices of Bacon

2 Slices of Cheddar cheese

2 Hamburger buns

Pinch of Salt

Pinch of Pepper

Condiments

Heavy-Duty Aluminum Foil

Preparation:

1. Wrap 2 pieces of bacon and 1 hamburger, and secure well with wooden picks.

2. Place each on different foils and fold the foils tightly around the burgers to make packets.

3. Transfer the packets to the heat and cook for 20 to 25 minutes.

4. Remove packets from the heat and open them gently.

5. Pour the cheese on the burger; then add condiments.

6. Enjoy.

BAKED BURGER BEANS

Ingredients:

1 Cup of Baked beans

1 Onion (diced)

8 oz. of Hamburger

½ Cup of Barbecue sauce

Breadcrumbs

Pinch of Salt

Pinch of Pepper

Heavy-Duty Aluminum Foil

Preparation:

1. Mix barbecue sauce, hamburger, onion, breadcrumbs, salt, and pepper in a bowl together.

2. Use your hand to form a patty from the hamburger and place it on a foil.

3. Pour the baked beans into the hamburger.

4. Fold the foil tightly to make a packet.

5. Transfer the packets to the heat and cook until the hamburger is well cooked or for 20 to 25 minutes.

6. Enjoy.

Veggie Steak

Ingredients:

½ Pound of Steak (cubed)

1 Potato (peeled, chunked)

½ Package of Onion soup

2 Tablespoons of Water

1 Tablespoon of Olive oil

¼ Cup of Mushrooms (sliced)

Pinch of Salt

Pinch of Pepper

Heavy-Duty Aluminum Foil

Preparation:

1. Blend the entire ingredients on a foil together.

2. Fold the foil tightly to make a packet, allowing room for the circulation of heat.

3. Transfer the packets to the heat and cook until the steak is well cooked and the vegetables are soft or for 20 to 25 minutes.

FOILED ORIENTAL STEAK

Ingredients:

16 oz. of Sirloin steak (cubed)

2 Red bell pepper (seeded, sliced)

1 Cup of Broccoli florets

¼ Cup of Parsley

4 Potatoes (sliced)

1 Onion (sliced)

2 Tablespoons of Garlic powder

¼ Cup of Olive oil

Pinch of Salt

Pinch of Pepper

Heavy-Duty Aluminum Foil

Preparation:

1. Combine entire ingredients in a bowl together.

2. Pour the mixture on a foil, and fold the foil tightly to make a packet.

3. Transfer the packets to the heat and cook until the veggies are well cooked or for 20 to 25 minutes.

4. Enjoy.

STEAK POTATOES & ASPARAGUS

Ingredients:

1 Ham Steak (pieces)

½ Cup of Alfredo sauce

8 Asparagus spears (pieces)

2 Red potatoes (pieces)

Heavy-Duty Aluminum Foil

Preparation:

1. Add the entire ingredients on a foil, and fold the foil tightly to make a packet.

2. Allow room for heat circulation in the packet.

3. Transfer the packets to the heat and cook until the asparagus is soft or for 15 to 20 minutes.

Sweet Potatoes Steak

Ingredients:

1 Ham Steak (chunked)

2 Potatoes (medium, cubed)

3 Rings of Pineapple (Chunked)

2 Tablespoons of Butter

2 Tablespoons of Brown sugar

Heavy-Duty Aluminum Foil

Preparation:

1. Add the entire ingredients on a foil, and fold the foil tightly to make a packet.

2. Allow room for heat circulation in the packet.

3. Transfer the packets to the heat and cook until the

potatoes and pineapple are soft or for 15 to 20 minutes.

4. Turn the packet to the other side and cook halfway.

5. Allow cooling before opening the packet.

CHEESY MEAT BREAD

Ingredients:

1 Ham Steak (sliced)

2 tablespoons of Butter

½ Loaf of Sourdough bread (sliced into 8 pieces)

4 Slices of Cheddar cheese

Heavy-Duty Aluminum Foil

Preparation:

1. Place the sliced bread on a foil.

2. Rub the butter in between bread pieces.

3. Add cheese on top of the buttered bread; then add meat on it, making 4 sandwiches.

4. Fold the foil tightly to make a packet.

5. Transfer the packets to the heat and cook until the cheese is melted or for 5 to 8 minutes.

CREAMY MUSHROOMS BEEF

Ingredients:

1 Pound of Beef (ground)

½ Cup of Mushrooms (sliced)

½ Cup of Corn niblets

1 Can of Cream of Mushrooms soup

½ Cup of Carrots (cut into coins)

Pinch of Salt

Pinch of Pepper

Heavy-Duty Aluminum Foil

Preparation:

1. Combine entire ingredients on a foil together.

2. Fold the foil tightly to make a packet.

3. Transfer the packets to the heat and cook until the veggies are soft or for 30 to 40 minutes.

Honey Potatoes & Pork Ribs

Ingredients:

½ Pound of Pork ribs (boneless)

1 Cup of Carrots (baby, halved)

4 Potatoes (halved)

¼ Cup of Honey

½ Teaspoon of Salt

¼ Cup of Barbecue sauce

1 Teaspoon of Cumin

Heavy-Duty Aluminum Foil

Preparation:

1. Combine honey, barbecue sauce, cumin, and salt in a bowl together.

2. Put the pork ribs, potatoes, and carrots on foil.

3. Pour the sauce over the ribs mix.

4. Fold the foil tightly to make a packet, allowing room for the circulation of heat.

5. Transfer the packets to the heat and grill until the pork ribs are cooked well and potatoes are soft or for 30 to 40 minutes.

Spiced Hot Dogs

Ingredients:

4 Hot dogs

1 onion (sliced)

1 Red pepper (sliced)

2 Teaspoons of Olive oil

1 Green pepper (sliced)

4 Hot dog buns

Mustard

Heavy-Duty Aluminum Foil

Preparation:

1. Divide the hot dogs into two and place them on two separate foils.

2. Divide also onions and peppers; then pour them on top of the hot dogs in the two foils.

3. Also repeat the process for olive oil.

4. Fold the foils tightly to make packets.

5. Transfer the packets to the heat and cook until the hot dogs are cooked well or for 30 to 40 minutes.

6. Remove from the heat and gently open the foils.

7. Put the hot, onion, and peppers on the buns.

8. Use mustard to season it.

ASIAN SWEET STEAK

Ingredients:

1 Pound of Steak (sliced)

¼ Cup of Soy sauce

2 Scallions (sliced)

2 Tablespoons of Rice vinegar

2 Teaspoons of Ginger (grated)

2 Tablespoons of Brown sugar

2 Teaspoons of Sesame oil

Red pepper

Heavy-Duty Aluminum Foil

Preparation:

1. Combine soy, vinegar, sesame oil, sugar, ginger, and red

pepper in a bowl together.

2. Put the scallion and steak on a foil.

3. Pour the soy sauce mix on top of the steak and scallion.

4. Fold the foil tightly to make a packet.

5. Transfer the packets to the heat and cook until the steaks are cooked well or for 15 to 20 minutes.

6. Allow cooling for few minutes before eating.

Lemony Steak & Asparagus

Ingredients:

1 Steak

4 Asparagus spears

1 Lemon (sliced)

1 Teaspoon of Olive oil

1 Tablespoon of Thyme

1 Teaspoon of Butter

Pinch of Salt

Pinch of Pepper

Heavy-Duty Aluminum Foil

Preparation:

1. Put the steak on a foil and surround it with asparagus.

2. Drizzle with thyme, salt, and pepper to taste.

3. Pour butter on the asparagus, and olive oil on every ingredient.

4. Fold the foil tightly to make a packet, allowing room for the circulation of heat.

5. Transfer the packets to the heat and cook until the steaks are cooked well or for 15 to 20 minutes.

6. Allow cooling for few minutes before opening the packet.

Meatballs with Potatoes

Ingredients:

1 Pound of Hamburger meat

4 Red potatoes (halved)

1 Cup of Carrots (chopped)

1 Onion (diced)

Ranch dressing

1 Tablespoon of Pepper

1 Tablespoon of Salt

Heavy-Duty Aluminum Foil

Preparation:

1. Blend salt and pepper with hamburger and make it into meatballs.

2. Put the meatballs on a foil; then place all the veggies around the meatballs.

3. Drizzle the ranch dressing on the veggies and meatballs.

4. Fold the foil tightly to make a packet, allowing room for the circulation of heat.

5. Transfer the packets to the heat and cook until the hamburger is cooked well or for 25 to 35 minutes.

6. Turn the packet halfway while cooking.

7. Gently open the packet.

Buttered Peach Pork

Ingredients:

2 Pork chops

2 Teaspoons of Balsamic vinegar

2 Tablespoons of Butter (melted)

2 Cups of Peach preserves

Heavy-Duty Aluminum Foil

Preparation:

1. Mix peach, butter, and vinegar in a bowl well.

2. Put the chops on a foil and use the peach mix to coat them.

3. Fold the foil tightly to make a packet.

4. Transfer the packets to the heat and cook until the pork chops are cooked well or for 25 to 35 minutes.

5. Remove the packet from the heat and gently open it after 5 minutes of cooling.

Spiced Sausage with Black Beans

Ingredients:

3/4 Pound of Sausage (smoked, sliced)

1 Carrot (peeled, diced)

1 Can of Black beans (drained, rinsed)

1 Shallot (diced)

1 Cup of Chicken broth

1 clove of Garlic (minced)

Pinch of Salt

Pinch of Pepper

Heavy-Duty Aluminum Foil

Preparation:

1. Add the entire ingredients on a foil well.

2. Rub salt and pepper on the mixture to taste.

3. Fold the foil tightly to make a packet, allowing room for the circulation of heat.

4. Transfer the packets to the heat and cook until the carrots are cooked well or for 25 to 35 minutes.

5. Enjoy.

Veggie & Steak

Ingredients:

2 Sirloin steaks

1 Cup of Mushrooms (sliced)

2 Potatoes (Shredded)

1 Onion (chopped)

1 Tablespoon of Olive oil

1 Cup of Green beans (halved)

Pinch of Salt

Pinch of Pepper

Heavy-Duty Aluminum Foil

Preparation:

1. Put the shredded potatoes on a foil.

2. Place onions, mushrooms, and green beans on top of the shredded potatoes.

3. Pour half of the olive oil on the veggies and use the remaining to rub steak with salt and pepper.

4. Put the steak on top of the vegetables.

5. Fold the foil tightly to make a packet.

6. Transfer the packets to the heat and cook until the vegetables are cooked well or for 30 to 45 minutes.

7. Enjoy.

Buttered Super Steak Packet

Ingredients:

1 Pound of Steak

1 cup of Onion soup mix

2 Potatoes (halved)

2 Stalks of Celery (cut into sticks)

¼ Cup of Margarine

2 Carrots (quartered)

1 Teaspoon of Salt

Heavy-Duty Aluminum Foil

Preparation:

1. Put the steak at the center of the foil and add onion soup mix.

2. Pour the entire vegetables on top of it.

3. Add margarine and sprinkle with salt.

4. Fold the foil tightly to make a packet, allowing room for the circulation of heat.

5. Transfer the packets to the heat and grill well or for 30 to 45 minutes.

Glazed Asian Ribs

Ingredients:

1 Pound of Baby back ribs

¼ Cup of Chili sauce

½ Tablespoon of Liquid smoke

½ Tablespoon of Honey

2 Tablespoons of Hoisin sauce

Pinch of Salt

Pinch of Cayenne salt

Heavy-Duty Aluminum Foil

Preparation:

1. Combine the entire ingredients except for ribs in a bowl well.

2. Coat the ribs with the mixture and place them in a single line on a foil.

3. Pour the remaining mix on top of the ribs.

4. Fold the foil tightly to make a packet, allowing room for the circulation of heat.

5. Transfer the packets to the heat and grill well or for 45 to 55 minutes.

6. Enjoy.

Mayo Ham with Cheese Buns

Ingredients:

6 oz. of Ham (diced, boneless)

½ Cup of Green onion (chopped)

¼ Cup of Cheddar cheese (shredded)

¼ Cup of Green olives (chopped)

1 Egg (hard-boiled, chopped)

¼ Cup of Chili sauce

1 ½ Tablespoons of Mayonnaise

3 Hamburger buns

Heavy-Duty Aluminum Foil

Preparation:

1. Mix the entire ingredients in a bowl together except buns

well.

2. Pour the mixture into the buns.

3. Place each bun on a separate foil.

4. Fold the foils tightly to make packets.

5. Transfer the packets to the heat and grill well or for 15 to 25 minutes.

6. Enjoy.

Chapter 6

FISH & SEAFOOD RECIPES

It is important to know that there are some meals from fish and seafood that can be cooked in the camp while on vacation with foiled packets. The only thing to remember is that these meals should be cooked well so as not to get sick due to undercooked food.

LEMONY BEER SHRIMP

Ingredients:

½ Pound of Shrimp (large, peeled, deveined)

½ Cup of Margarine

1 Shallot (sliced)

3 Tablespoons of Lemon juice

½ Can of Beer

1 clove of Garlic

Pinch of Salt

Pinch of Pepper

Heavy-Duty Aluminum Foil

Preparation:

1. Combine the entire ingredients on a foil.

2. Fold the foil tightly to make a packet.

3. Transfer the packets to the heat and cook until the shrimps are well cooked or for 30 to 40 minutes.

4. Enjoy.

Seasoned Lemony Catfish

Ingredients:

2 Catfish fillets

1 Cup of Green and Red bell peppers (chopped)

1 Can of Corn

1 Tablespoon of Cajun seasoning

2 Tablespoons of Olive oil

2 Jalapeno pepper (chopped)

2 Tablespoons of Lime juice

2 Teaspoons of Cilantro (chopped)

Heavy-Duty Aluminum Foil

Preparation:

1. Lay each fillet on a different foil.

2. Rub both fillets with half a portion of seasoning.

3. Mix the remaining ingredient with the seasoning well.

4. Use a spoon to pour the mixture on each fillet.

5. Fold the foils tightly to make packets, allowing room for the circulation of heat.

6. Transfer the packets to the heat and cook until the catfishes are well cooked or for 30 to 40 minutes.

7. Carefully open the packets and garnish them with cilantro.

Wine & Buttered Sausage

Ingredients:

¾ Pound of Clams

¼ Pound of Sausage (sliced)

1 ½ Tablespoons of Butter

2 cloves of Garlic (sliced)

1 1/2 Tablespoons of Butter

¾ Cup of White Wine

1 ½ Tablespoons of Olive oil

Pinch of Salt

Pinch of Black pepper

Heavy-Duty Aluminum Foil

Preparation:

1. Put the entire ingredients on foil.

2. Fold the foils tightly to make packets, allowing room for the circulation of heat.

3. Transfer the packet to the heat and cook until they are well cooked or for 20 to 30 minutes.

4. Enjoy.

LEMONY MILKY SHRIMPS

Ingredients:

1 Pound of Shrimp (peeled, deveined)

¼ Cup of Lime juice

1 Cup of Coconut milk

¼ Cup of Coconut (shredded)

Heavy-Duty Aluminum Foil

Preparation:

1. Put the entire ingredients on foil.

2. Fold the foil tightly to make a packet.

3. Transfer the packet to the heat and cook until the shrimps are well cooked or for 15 to 20 minutes.

4. Enjoy.

Assorted Cod Fillet

Ingredients:

2 Cod fillets

2 cloves of Garlic (chopped)

10 Cherry tomatoes

10 Olives

2 Teaspoons of Basil (chopped)

1 Cup of Chicken broth

¼ Cup of Olive oil

2 Teaspoons of Mint (chopped)

2 Teaspoons of Oregano

Heavy-Duty Aluminum Foil

Preparation:

1. Lay the cods on a foil.

2. Surround the fillets with olives and tomatoes

3. Fold the foil tightly to make a packet, allowing room for the circulation of heat, and then open the top side.

4. Pour in the remaining ingredients and cover the side opened.

3. Transfer the packet to the heat and cook until the fillets and tomatoes are well cooked or for 20 to 35 minutes.

5. Serve and enjoy while hot.

Cheesy Sriracha Cod

Ingredients:

1 Pound of Cod

2 Flour Tortilla

1/3 Cup of Cabbage (shredded)

1/3 Cup of Italian seasoning

2 Tablespoons of Lime juice (wedged)

Sriracha Sauce

Cheddar Cheese

Sour cream

Heavy-Duty Aluminum Foil

Preparation:

1. Put the cod on a foil.

2. Rub the Italian seasoning on the fish.

3. Drizzle the lime juice on it.

4. Fold the foil tightly to make a packet.

5. Transfer the packet to the heat and cook until the fishes are well cooked or for 20 to 30 minutes.

6. Remove the packet from the heat and carefully open it.

7. Break the cod into bits and lay it on the tortillas.

8. Then add cheese, cabbage, sour cream, and Sriracha Sauce.

9. Enjoy.

PARSLEY FLAVOURED FISH

Ingredients:

2 Fillets

¼ Cup of Butter

2 Tablespoons of Parsley (chopped)

1 Onion (chopped)

1 Lemon (halved)

Pinch of Salt

Pinch of Pepper

Heavy-Duty Aluminum Foil

Preparation:

1. Put the fillets on the foil.

2. Add onions, butter, parsley, salt, and pepper.

3. Fold the foil tightly to make a packet.

4. Squeeze the halved lime on the fillets on the foil.

5. Fold the foil tightly to make a packet.

6. Transfer the packet to the heat and cook until the fishes are well cooked or for 20 to 25 minutes.

7. Enjoy.

SPICED LEMONY TROUT

Ingredients:

2 Trout fillets

2 Green onions

1 Lemon (wedged)

¼ Cup of Butter

2 Sprigs of Thyme

Pinch of Salt

Pinch of Pepper

Heavy-Duty Aluminum Foil

Preparation:

1. Lay the fillets on the foil.

2. Squeeze the halved lime on the fillets on the foil.

3. Surround the remaining lemon wedge around the fillets.

4. Put the butter on top of the fillets.

5. Then sprinkle onions and thyme on the fillets.

6. Put salt and pepper to taste.

7. Fold the foil tightly to make a packet.

6. Transfer the packet to the heat and cook until the fishes are well cooked or for 10 to 15 minutes.

Buttered Lemony Lobster

Ingredients:

1 Lobster tail (halved, shelled)

¼ Cup of Parsley (chopped)

¼ Cup of Butter

1 Clove of Garlic (medium, chopped)

1 Teaspoon of Lemon juice

Pinch of Salt

Pinch of Pepper

Heavy-Duty Aluminum Foil

Preparation:

1. Put the entire ingredients on foil.

2. Fold the foil tightly to make a packet.

3. Transfer the packet to the heat and cook until the lobster tails are well cooked or for 10 to 15 minutes.

4. Add salt and pepper to season it.

5. Enjoy.

PARSLEY MUSSELS SAUCE

Ingredients:

1 Pound of Mussels (fresh)

1 Cup of White wine

1 Stick of Butter (unsalted)

½ Cup of Lemon juice

1 Cup of Parsley (chopped)

2 cloves of Garlic (minced)

2 Tablespoons of Tabasco sauce

Heavy-Duty Aluminum Foil

Preparation:

1. Put the mussels on a foil.

2. Wrap the foil on the mussels to make a packet, and open the top side.

3. Pour the remaining ingredients into the packet and cover it up, and allow room for the circulation of heat.

4. Transfer the packet to the heat and cook until they are well cooked or for 10 to 15 minutes.

5. Enjoy.

CITRUS SHRIMP

Ingredients:

3 Pound of Shrimp (peeled, deveined)

1 clove of Garlic (minced)

3 Oranges (Juiced)

1 Teaspoon of Zest

2 Teaspoons of Olive oil

Pinch of Salt

Pinch of Pepper

Heavy-Duty Aluminum Foil

Preparation:

1. Pour the orange juice into a sealable plastic bag.

2. Then stir in garlic, orange zest, and olive oil in the bag.

3. Shake the bag well and then add shrimp.

4. Shake the contents in the bag until the shrimps are well coated.

5. Put the coated shrimps on the foil; then pour the remaining mix in the bag on the shrimps.

6. Season it with salt and pepper.

7. Fold the foil tightly to make a packet.

8. Transfer the packet to the heat and cook the shrimps until they are well cooked or for 10 to 15 minutes.

Seasoned Chicken & Smoked Shrimp

Ingredients:

1 Chicken breast (boneless, skinless, boiled, cubed)

4 oz. of Shrimp (jumbo, peeled, deveined)

1 Sausage (smoked, sliced)

1 Tomato (medium, diced)

½ Cup of Brown sugar

1 Green bell pepper (diced)

1 Red bell pepper (diced)

1 Stick of Celery (diced)

½ Cup of Onions (diced)

1 Bay leaf

1 Tablespoon of Cajun seasoning

2 Teaspoons of Garlic powder

1 Tablespoon of Hot sauce

Heavy-Duty Aluminum Foil

Preparation:

1. Blend the entire ingredients in a bowl well.

2. Fold the foil tightly to make a packet, allowing room for the circulation of heat.

3. Transfer the packet to the heat and cook the shrimps, chicken, and vegetables until they are well cooked or for 20 to 25 minutes.

4. Open the packets gently and season them with salt and pepper.

5. Enjoy.

SPICED SHRIMPS

Ingredients:

8 Shrimps (jumbo, peeled, deveined)

½ Bell pepper (seeded, sliced)

½ Onion (chopped)

1 Flour Tortilla

2 Tablespoons of Olive oil

½ Bell pepper (seeded, sliced)

Pinch of Paprika

Pinch of Cayenne pepper

Pinch of Cumin

Salsa

Cheese

Heavy-Duty Aluminum Foil

Preparation:

1. Combine paprika, olive oil, cayenne pepper, and cumin in a bowl thoroughly.

2. Stir in onion, bell pepper, and shrimp in the mixture well.

3. Stir until the shrimp are well coated.

4. Pour the mixture on a foil, and fold the foil tightly to make a packet.

5. Transfer the packet to the heat and cook the shrimps until they are well cooked or for 20 to 25 minutes.

6. Put the mixture on the tortilla, and garnish it with cheese and salsa.

7. Enjoy.

Lemony Buttered Shrimp

Ingredients:

1 Pound of Shrimp (peeled, deveined)

1 Cup of Parsley (chopped)

1 Cup of Butter

2 Tablespoons of Lemon juice

2 cloves of Garlic (minced)

Pinch of Salt

Pinch of Pepper

Heavy-Duty Aluminum Foil

Preparation:

1. Put the entire ingredients on a foil, and drizzle lemon juice on the mixture.

2. Fold the foil tightly to make a packet.

3. Transfer the packet to the heat and cook the shrimps until they are well cooked or for 10 to 15 minutes.

4. Season the shrimp with salt and pepper.

5. Enjoy.

Easy Grilled Salmon

Ingredients:

2 Salmon steak

¼ Cup of Butter

1 Lemon (sliced)

Pinch of Salt

Pinch of Black Pepper

Heavy-Duty Aluminum Foil

Preparation:

1. Put the lemon slices on the foil.

2. Put the salmon on top of the lemon, and pour the butter on top of the salmon.

3. Season it with salt and black pepper.

4. Fold the foil tightly to make a packet.

5. Transfer the packet to the heat and cook the salmons until they are well cooked or for 30 to 35 minutes.

GINGERED SWORDFISH STEAK

Ingredients:

2 Swordfishes

2 Carrots (cut into strips)

4 Shallots (chopped)

2 Tablespoons of Butter

2 Teaspoons of Lemon juice

2 Teaspoons of Teriyaki sauce

2 Teaspoons of Ginger root (grated)

Heavy-Duty Aluminum Foil

Preparation:

1. Combine the entire ingredients on a foil.

2. Fold the foil tightly to make a packet.

3. Transfer the packet to the heat and cook the fish and carrots until they are well cooked or for 30 to 45 minutes.

4. Enjoy.

EASY SALMON & TERIYAKI SAUCE

Ingredients:

2 Salmon fillets

2 Green bell peppers (sliced)

1 Onion (sliced)

2 Red bell peppers (sliced)

1 Cup of teriyaki sauce

Heavy-Duty Aluminum Foil

Preparation:

1. Put the salmon on a foil.

2. Place the veggies around the fish.

3. Fold the foil tightly to make a packet, allowing room for the circulation of heat.

4. Transfer the packet to the heat and cook the salmon and vegetables until they are well cooked or for 25 to 35 minutes.

5. Enjoy.

Amazing Zucchini Tilapia

Ingredients:

2 Tilapia fillets (skinless)

2 Zucchini (sliced)

2 cloves of Garlic (chopped)

2 Tablespoons of Olive oil

1 Tomato (diced)

1 Teaspoon of Oregano

2 Tablespoons of Basil leaves (chopped)

Pinch of Salt

Pinch of Pepper

Heavy-Duty Aluminum Foil

Preparation:

1. Lay each zucchini and tilapia on two different foils.

2. Then put the other zucchini and tilapia on top of the one on the foils.

3. Put the tomato on them and drizzle olive oil on them.

4. Then add oregano, garlic, basil leaves, salt, and pepper.

5. Fold the foils tightly to make packets, allowing room for the circulation of heat.

6. Transfer the packet to the heat and cook the tilapia and zucchini until they are well cooked or for 25 to 35 minutes.

Creamy Tuna Buns

Ingredients:

5 oz. of Tuna

½ Cup of Mozzarella cheese

¼ Cup of Mayonnaise

½ Cup of Celery (chopped)

1 Tablespoon of Onion (grated)

3 Hamburger buns

Heavy-Duty Aluminum Foil

Preparation:

1. Blend the entire ingredients in a bowl well, except the buns.

2. Pour the mix on the buns on the foil.

3. Fold the foils tightly to make packets.

4. Transfer the packet to the heat and cook the tilapia and zucchini until they are well cooked or for 10 to 15 minutes.

Chapter 7

DESSERT & ASSORTED RECIPES

The set of recipes in this section does not fall into any particular categories of meals. But, believe me, they are what will keep in check your cravings and pangs of hunger in between meals.

CHOCOLATE BANANA

Ingredients:

2 Bananas

Chocolate bits

Marshmallow

Graham crackers (crumbled)

Heavy-Duty Aluminum Foil

Preparation:

1. Cut the bananas in half lengthwise with the peels.

2. Place the bananas on a foil and add marshmallows and chocolate bits inside it.

3. Pour the crackers crumbs on top of the bananas.

4. Fold the foil tightly to make a packet.

5. Transfer the packets to the heat and cook until the chocolate bits have melted or for 10 to 15 minutes.

Sweet Milky Oatmeal

Ingredients:

3 Cups of Instant oatmeal

¾ Cup of Milk (powder)

¾ Cup of Water

¼ Cup of Brown sugar

1 ½ Teaspoons of Cinnamon

Heavy-Duty Aluminum Foil

Preparation:

1. Combine the entire ingredients on a foil well.

2. Fold the foil tightly to make a packet.

3. Transfer the packets to the heat and cook until the oatmeal is thick or for 10 to 15 minutes.

4. Carefully open the packet and allow resting for few minutes before eating.

5. Enjoy.

Spiced Cheesy Salsa

Ingredients:

1 Cup of Cream cheese

1 Teaspoon of Onion (chopped)

1 Teaspoon of Basil

1 Cup of Velveeta cheese

1 Green onion (chopped)

1 Cup of Salsa

1 Teaspoon of Oregano

1 Teaspoon of Paprika

Heavy-Duty Aluminum Foil

Preparation:

1. Put the cream cheese on a foil and place the crumble

Velveeta on top of the cream cheese.

2. Then add paprika, oregano, and basil to the cheeses.

3. Fold the foil tightly to make a packet.

4. Transfer the packets to the heat and cook until the cheeses are melted or for 7 to 10 minutes.

5. Open the packet gently and stir it well.

6. Pour in green onion and salsa.

7. Serve with your favorite dipping.

Marinated Cheese Pizza

Ingredients:

10 Sticks of Pizza crust

1 Tablespoon of Parmesan cheese

½ Cup of Cheddar cheese

1 Tablespoon of Olive oil

½ Cup of Marinara sauce

1 Tablespoon of Garlic (powder)

Heavy-Duty Aluminum Foil

Preparation:

1. Put the crusts on a foil, brush them with olive oil.

2. Season them with garlic and sprinkle with cheese.

3. Fold the foil tightly to make a packet.

4. Transfer the packets to the heat and cook until the dough is baked and cheeses are melted or for 15 to 20 minutes.

5. Enjoy it with marinara sauce and your favorite dipping.

Cheesy Chili French Fries

Ingredients:

¼ Package of French fries

½ Cup of Chili con carne

½ Cup of Mozzarella

Pinch of Salt

Pinch of Pepper

Heavy-Duty Aluminum Foil

Preparation:

1. Put the French fries on a foil.

2. Add salt and pepper to the fries.

3. Fold the foil tightly to make a packet.

5. Put the chili in another foil.

6. Top it with cheese and fold the foil tightly to make a packet

7. Transfer the packets to the heat and cook until the fries are cooked well or for 15 to 20 minutes.

8. Wait for few minutes for the packet to cool.

9. Top the Chili packet on top of the fries, and enjoy.

Sweet Spiced Pineapple Doughnut

Ingredients:

1 Can of Pineapple chunks

2 Teaspoons of Brown sugar

1 Teaspoon of Olive oil

2 Cake doughnuts (plain)

2 Teaspoons of Butter

2 Teaspoons of Cinnamon

Heavy-Duty Aluminum Foil

Preparation:

1. Rub the foil with olive oil.

2. Put the pineapple chunks on the foil.

3. Divide the cake and put it on the foil.

4. Then add sugar, butter, and cinnamon over it.

5. Fold the foil tightly to make a packet.

6. Transfer the packets to the heat and cook until the butter is melted and pineapple is cooked well or for 15 to 20 minutes.

7. Pour whipped cream to the top of it if desired.

Quick Cheesy Milky Mac

Ingredients:

1 Cup of Macaroni (cooked)

1 Cup of Cheddar cheese

½ Cup of Milk

2 Tablespoons Butter

Pinch of Salt

Pinch of Pepper

Heavy-Duty Aluminum Foil

Preparation:

1. Combine the entire ingredients on a foil together.

2. Fold the foil tightly to make a packet.

3. Transfer the packets to the heat and cook until the cheese is melted or for 15 to 20 minutes.

4. Open the packet carefully and stir before eating.

Cinnamon Marshmallow Peach

Ingredients:

2 Peaches (halved, pitted)

1 Teaspoon of Cinnamon

Mini Marshmallow

2 Teaspoons of Butter

Heavy-Duty Aluminum Foil

Preparation:

1. Put the peaches on the foil making sure the sides are up.

2. Pour the butter into the pitted peaches, and fill them up with marshmallows.

3. Put cinnamon on top and close the peaches to make them whole again.

4. Fold the foil tightly to make a packet.

5. Transfer the packets to the heat and cook until the marshmallow begins to melt or for 5 to 10 minutes.

6. Allow it to cool before eating.

Quick Fruit Pies

Ingredients:

2 Pie Crusts (mini)

1 Can of Fruit pie filling

Heavy-Duty Aluminum Foil

Preparation:

1. Put the pie crusts on a foil.

2. Add pie filling to the pie crust.

3. Fold the foil tightly to make a packet.

4. Transfer the packet to the heat, making sure it stands upright.

5. Cook until filling is well cooked or for 5 to 10 minutes.

6. Enjoy.

CHEESY BEANS TORTILLAS

Ingredients:

1 Cup of Tortilla chips

½ Cup of Beans (refried)

¼ Cup of Salsa

1 Cup of American Blend cheese

Heavy-Duty Aluminum Foil

Preparation:

1. Put the tortilla on a foil.

2. Surround the tortilla chips with beans.

3. Fold the foil tightly to make a packet, and poke it severally at the top.

4. Transfer the packets to the heat and cook until the cheese

is melted and the beans are heated through or for 5 to 10 minutes.

5. Carefully open the packet and top it with salsa and cheese.

6. Serve while hot.

Caramelized Orange Cinnamon Rolls

Ingredients:

2 Oranges

¼ Cup of Caramel

4 Rolls of Cinnamon

Heavy-Duty Aluminum Foil

Preparation:

1. Cut the oranges and remove the flesh parts, to have hollow shells.

2. Put each cinnamon in a shell.

3. Divide the shells into two and place each portion on a foil making two foils.

4. Fold the foils tightly to make packets.

5. Transfer the packets to the heat and cook until the cinnamon begins to brown or for 10 to 15 minutes.

6. Remove them from the heat and carefully open them.

7. Pour on them caramel and serve while warm.

Quick Cheese Tortilla

Ingredients:

1 Cup of Mexican blend cheese (shredded)

2 Flour of tortilla

Heavy-Duty Aluminum Foil

Preparation:

1. Pour the cheese on each tortilla and fold it in half.

2. Place each tortilla on a different foil.

3. Fold the foils tightly to make packets.

4. Transfer the packets to the heat and cook until the cheese is melted or for 10 to 15 minutes.

Peanut Grilled Tortilla

Ingredients:

2 Flour of Tortilla

Mini Marshmallows

2 Tablespoons of Peanut butter

Chocolate chips

Heavy-Duty Aluminum Foil

Preparation:

1. Rub the butter on the tortilla, add chocolate, and marshmallows as you want on it.

2. Roll the tortillas up to look like a burrito.

3. Fold the foil tightly to make a packet.

4. Transfer the packets to the heat and cook until chocolate

and marshmallow are melted or for 10 to 15 minutes.

5. Allow it to cool and enjoy.

Super Delight Marshmallow Cone

Ingredients:

2 Waffle cones

Mini Marshmallows

Peanut butter

Chocolate chips

Mini Pretzels

Heavy-Duty Aluminum Foil

Preparation:

1. Pour marshmallows, mini-pretzels, chocolate chips, and peanuts into the cones.

2. Fold the foil tightly to make a packet.

3. Transfer the packet to the heat and cook until chocolate

and marshmallow are melted or for 7 to 10 minutes.

4. Open and allow for a few minutes before eating.

Sweet Glazed Pineapple

Ingredients:

1 Pineapple (peeled, cored, and cut into rings)

¼ Cup of Honey

4 Tablespoons of Dark rum

Heavy-Duty Aluminum Foil

Preparation:

1. Put the pineapple on the foil, and pour rum and honey over it.

2. Fold the foil tightly to make a packet.

3. Transfer the packet to the heat and cook until chocolate and marshmallow are melted or for 15 to 20 minutes.

4. Serve the glazed pineapple with ham.

CONCLUSION

I hope you enjoyed reading this book!

Don't you think you should get rid of attending to domestic chores like washing silverware and cleaning utensils while on an outdoor camp?

But how will you feel when you have at your disposal easy, quick, and delicious meals that either campfire or grill will cook using aluminum foil?

Among what you want to experience and enjoy is the delicious smoky flavor of meals cooked over fire.

This book is about easily prepared meals you can cook while camping that will not take your time, less expensive, and with easy to get ingredients.

Foil packets meals are gotten through a kind of cooking method that will make you enjoy your adventure as you won't have to worry about washing silverware, giving you more time to enjoy your stay in the park.

If you enjoyed reading the book and have tried the recipes included, let us know.

Thank You.

INTERNAL TEMPERATURE COOKING CHARTS

Beef, Lamb, Pork, Veal, Roasts, Ham

Rare	120-130°F
Rare Medium	130-135°F
Medium	135-145°F
Medium Well	145-155°F
Well Cooked	155F and above

Pork Ribs

Well Cooked	190-205°F

Poultry

Well Cooked	Minimum 165°F

Fish

Well Cooked	Minimum 135°F

COOKING CONVERSION CHARTS

Measuring Equivalent Chart

Type	Metric	Imperial	Imperial
Weight	28g	1 oz.	
	0.45kg	1 Pound	16 oz.
Volume	5 ml	1 Teaspoon	
	10 ml	1 Desert Spoon	2 Teaspoons
	15 ml	1 Tablespoon	3 Teaspoons
	20 ml	1 Australian Tablespoon	4 Teaspoons
	30 ml	1 Fluid ounce	2 Tablespoons
	240 ml	1 Cup	16 Tablespoons
	240 ml	1 Cup	8 Fluid ounces
	470 ml	1 Pint	2 Cups
	0.95 l	1 Pint	2 Cups

	3.8 l	1 Gallon	4 Quarts
Length	2.54 cm	1 Inch	

Oven Temperature Equivalent Chart

T°F	T°C
220	100
225	110
250	120
275	140
300	150
325	160
350	180
375	190

400	200
425	220
450	230
475	250
500	260